Drug Calculation Workbook

For Healthcare Professionals

John England

Table of Contents

Disclaimer..4

Preface...5

Introduction..7

Abbreviations...10

Unit Conversions...15

Body Mass Index...22

Body Surface Area..30

Tablet Dosages..39

Ampoule Dosages...47

Drip Rates..56

Pumped Infusions...65

Displacement Volume..73

W/V Drug Concentration..................................83

Dilutions...92

Test One...104

Test two – with answers..................................112

Drug Calculation Workbook

Test two - questions only 121

Test Three – with answers 124

Test three – questions only 132

Books by John England 135

Favourite Quotes 137

Disclaimer

The author has made every effort to ensure that the contents of this book are correct, error free, and a reasonable representation of the design goal, which is to present worked examples of a selection of drug calculation problems. This body of work should be regarded as a text book for learning purposes, and not a clinical manual.

The author accepts no responsibility or liability for damages caused by any erroneous contents of this book and, in all situations, recommends that professional guidelines, national policies, and direction from suitably qualified medical staff, take precedence over the information contained herein.

All rights reserved. The contents of this book may not be duplicated or distributed in any form, without written permission from the author.

Preface

Drug Calculation Workbook provides the reader with further examples of drug calculation problems, using metric and other S.I. units, as described and discussed in the accompanying textbook "**Basic Drug Calculations**" (*John England, Amazon Publishing*).

Aimed at all healthcare professionals, such as nurses, doctors, paramedics, and perioperative technicians and practitioners, the subject matter is highly relevant, and addresses the need to practise typical drug calculation problems, from the most basic, up to problems which might be considered at an intermediate level of difficulty, and of a type likely to be encountered on interview drug calculation assessment tests.

More advanced types of drug calculation, such as molar measurements, are not addressed here. Instead, they can be found in my other publication - **"Pass Your Drug Calculation Test"** (*John England, Amazon Publishing*).

To allow the reader to focus on the core component of a drug dosage calculation – the calculation itself - rather than complicate the problem with matters of pharmacology, drug names are not given. Instead, drugs are anonymised with letters of the alphabet, such as "drug X" and "drug A".

Introduction

Drug Calculation Workbook divides drug calculation problem types into nine categories, and includes questions posed for each of the categories, with worked solutions describing the discrete steps in solving the particular problems. The sections on Body Mass Index and Body Surface Area, although not directly concerning drug calculations, are part of the suite of calculations which influence drug dosages, so they are included - for completeness.

The calculation categories include:

- Unit conversions
- Body Mass Index
- Body Surface Area
- Tablet and Ampoule dosages

- Giving set drip rates
- Pumped infusions
- Displacement volumes
- Drug Concentrations
- Concentration Dilutions

To consolidate the above calculation types, they are followed by three sample tests, again with worked solutions, with the first test being the simplest, the second slightly more difficult, and the third test being more difficult than the second. Note that, to reflect the different ways in which drug calculation problems might be posed, the wording and style of questions are presented in a variety of ways. Also note that the terms "mass" and "weight" are used interchangeably, as they are in practice.

For those readers who have appropriate mathematical skills, it may only be necessary to study the contents of the book once and, thereafter, use it as a reference or quick revision tool.

For those whose mathematical skills are not so strong, the key to mastering the given drug calculation problems is to repeatedly and regularly copy out the questions and solutions because, by doing so, their familiarity can produce comprehension.

By following the old adage of "practice-practice-practice", the reader can expect to gain confidence in one of the most important functions of healthcare delivery, which is the accurate calculation of drug dosages.

Abbreviations

One of the most common causes of drug calculation error, for even the most competent mathematicians, is to misread or confuse units of discrimination, such as milligrams and micrograms, often because the units are abbreviated, and unclear. The commonly used unit types, and their abbreviations - duplicated from **Basic Drug Calculations** (*John England, Amazon Publishing*) - are as follows:

Unit abbreviations

Unit	Abbreviation
Litre	L or l
Millilitre	ml

Microlitre	**microlitre**
Mole	**mol**
Millimole	**mmol**
Micromole	**micromol**
Gram	**g**
Milligram	**mg**
Microgram	**microgram**
Nanogram	**nanogram**

Notice that the smaller units should not be abbreviated, instead, they should be written out in full. By doing so, the probability of confusing different units is minimised.

Prefixes

The S.I. (Système International d'Unités) unit prefixes are as follows:

Drug Calculation Workbook

Prefix	Factor
Peta	1,000,000,000,000,000
Tera	1,000,000,000,000
Giga	1,000,000,000
Mega	1,000,000
Kilo	1,000
Hecto	100
Deka	10
Deci	1 divided by 10
Centi	1 divided by 100
Milli	1 divided by 1,000
Micro	1 divided by 1,000,000
Nano	1 divided by 1,000,000,000
Pico	1 divided by 1,000,000,000,000

With respect to safety, understanding the above lists of abbreviations and unit discriminants is mandatory, so refer to them frequently, because using them correctly is required practise, and promotes safety.

Plurals

When discussing a unit type, such as microgram, in the plural, it is normal to add the "s" suffix; for example, a written instruction might declare that dosages should be measured in "micrograms". When, on the other hand, a specific value is given, the "s" should be omitted. For example, write "25 microgram", and not "25 micrograms".

Spacing

Another commonly made error, when denoting unit abbreviations, is to concatenate the value and abbreviation, as in "25ml", or "25mls". The correct format, as specified by many pharmacology governing bodies, is to omit the "s", and leave a space between the number and abbreviation; so the above volume should be written "25 ml" (NOT 25 c.c.).

Again, the purpose of such protocols is to promote clarity, and the purpose of clarity is to minimise errors of interpretation.

Note: Another acceptable abbreviation, because it cannot be easily confused for anything else, is **gtt**, which denotes a giving set's drops per ml.

Unit Conversions

When dealing with calculations, values should always be converted to the same measurement system and domain, such as converting imperial pounds to kilograms, and ensuring variables measured in micrograms, for example, are not included in the same calculation as variables measured in milligrams.

Another recommended practice is to avoid expressing variables in decimals and, instead, convert the value to a smaller type; for example, instead of using 0.0475 mg, multiply by 1,000 to form 47.5 microgram.

To be fully proficient at unit conversions, specifically in the metric system, some basic rules of unit division and discrimination must be mastered. Specifically, with respect to prefixes for canonical units, such as the kilogram or litre.

Unit Conversion Examples

Conversion Example 1

Convert 6' 1" to its metric equivalent.

~ Solution ~

Step 1: Convert 6' to inches: 6 * 12 = 72 inch.

Step 2: Add 1 = 73 inch.

Step 3: 1 inch = 2.5 cm, so 73 * 2.5 = 182.5 cm.

Answer: 182.5 cm (1.825 m).

Conversion Example 2

How many centilitres are there in one decilitre?

~ Solution ~

Step 1: One centilitre is 1 litre/100 = 10 ml.

Step 2: One decilitre is 1 litre/10 = 100 ml.

Step 3: 100/10 = 10 centilitre to 1 decilitre.

Answer: 10 centilitre = 1 decilitre.

Conversion Example 3

Convert 0.033 g to micrograms.

~ *Solution* ~

Step 1: Remind yourself that a gram is composed of 1,000 milligram, and 1 milligram is composed of 1,000 microgram.

Step 2: Convert 0.033 g to mg: 0.033 * 1,000 = 33 mg.

Step 3: Convert 33 mg to microgram: 33 * 1,000 33,000.

Answer: 0.033 g = 33,000 microgram.

Conversion Example 4

Convert 45,500 nanogram to mg (milligrams).

~ Solution ~

Step 1: Remind yourself that 1 mg = 1,000 microgram, and 1 microgram is composed of 1,000 nanogram.

Step 2: Convert nanogram to microgram: 45,500/1,000 = 45.5 microgram.

Step 3: Convert to mg: 45.5/1,000 = 0.0455 mg.

Answer: 0.0455 mg.

Conversion Example 5

Add 450 mg to 2.4 g.

~ Solution ~

Step 1: Convert to a common unit by changing the milligram value to grams; 450 mg/1,000 = 0.45 g.

Step 2: Add 0.45 g to 2.4 g = 2.85 g.

Answer: 2.85 g.

Drug Calculation Workbook

Conversion Example 6

Add 70 microgram to 0.35 mg and 2.1 mg.

~ Solution ~

Step 1: Convert 70 microgram to mg: 70/1,000 = 0.07 mg.

Step 2: Add 0.07, 0.35, and 2.1 = 2.52 mg.

Answer: 2.52 mg.

Conversion Example 7

Subtract 335 microgram from 2.2 mg.

~ Solution ~

Step 1: Convert mg to microgram: 2.2 * 1,000 = 2,200 microgram.

Step 2: Subtract 335 from 2,200 = 1,865 microgram.

Step 3: Convert 1,865 microgram to mg: 1,865/1,000 =

1.865 mg.

Answer: 1.865 mg.

Conversion Example 8

Subtract 0.15 L (litre) from 600 ml.

~ Solution ~

Step 1: Convert 0.15 L to ml: 0.15 * 1,000 = 150 ml.

Step 2: Subtract 150 from 600 ml = 450 ml.

Answer: 450 ml.

Conversion Example 9

Add 400 ml to 0.8 L (litre).

~ Solution ~

Step 1: Convert 0.8 L to ml: 0.8 * 1,000 = 800 ml.

Step 2: Add 800 to 400 = 1,200 ml.

Step 3: Convert ml to L: 1,200/1,000 = 1.2 L.

Answer: 1.2 litre.

Conversion Example 10

Multiply 90 nanogram by 12.

~ Solution ~

Step 1: 90 * 12 = 1,080 nanogram.

Step 2: Convert to microgram: 1,080/1,000 = 1.08 microgram.

Answer: 1.08 microgram.

Body Mass Index

BMI is an indirect ratio of a person's mass (weight) to their height, and is used as an indication of how underweight or overweight a patient is. The BMI value can be determined by dividing body weight (kg) by the square of the height (height^2), in metres.

$$BMI = weight / (height * height)$$

A "normal" BMI is considered to be between 18.5 and 25, with obesity classed at values of 30 or over.

<u>Note</u>: (1) Rounding up to one decimal place gives an acceptable degree of accuracy. (2) Terminology and abbreviations have been mixed – for variety. (3) "Mass" is usually, but incorrectly, described as "weight", so both terms will be used here.

Drug Calculation Workbook

Body Mass Index Examples

BMI Example 1

Determine the BMI for a patient who weighs 56 kg, and has a height of 5 foot 4 inch. (BMI = weight/height^2)

~ Solution ~

Step 1: Convert 5 feet to inches; 5*12 = 60.

Step 2: Add 60 and 4 = 64 inch.

Step 3: Recall that 1 inch is 2.5 cm.

Step 4: Convert the 64 inch to metric; 64 * 2.5 = 160 cm.

Step 5: Convert 160 cm to metres; 160/100 = 1.6 m.

Step 6: Square the height; 1.6 * 1.6 = **2.56**.

Step 7: Divide body weight (mass) by the squared height; 56/2.56 = 21.875, rounded to 21.9.

Answer: BMI = 21.9.

BMI Example 2

Determine the BMI for a patient who weighs 94 kg, and has a height of 1.8 metre. (BMI = weight/height^2).

~ Solution ~

Step 1: Square the height; 1.8 * 1.8 = 3.24.

Step 2: Divide weight by height^2; 94/3.24 = 29.15.

Answer: BMI = 29.

BMI Example 3

Determine the BMI for a patient who weighs 42 kg, and has a height of 165 cm (BMI = weight/height^2).

~ Solution ~

Step 1: Convert 165 cm to metres; 165/100 = 1.65 m.

Step 2: Square the height; 1.65 * 1.65 = 2.7.

Step 3: Weight/height^2; 42/2.7 = 15.5.

Answer: BMI = 15.5.

BMI Example 4

Determine the BMI for a patient who weighs 116 kg, and has a height of 1.9 m (BMI = weight/height^2).

~ Solution ~

Step 1: Height^2; 1.9 * 1.9 = 3.61.

Step 2: Weight/height^2; 116/3.61 = 32.1.

Answer: BMI = 32.1.

BMI Example 5

Determine the BMI for a patient whose body mass is 119 pounds, and has a height of 1.75 metre (BMI = mass/height^2).

~ Solution ~

Step 1: Convert 119 lb to kg; 119/2.2 = **54 kg**.

Step 2: Height^2; 1.75 * 1.75 = 3.06.

Step 3: Weight/height^2; 54/3.06 = 17.4.

Answer: BMI = 17.6.

BMI Example 6

Determine the BMI for a patient who has a height of 2.1 m, and weighs 71 kg (BMI = weight/height^2).

~ Solution ~

Step 1: Height^2 is 2.1 * 2.1 = 4.4.

Step 2: Weight/height^2 71/4.4 = 16.1.

Answer: BMI = 16.1.

BMI Example 7

Determine the BMI for a patient who weighs 48 kg, and has a height of 1.86 metre (BMI = weight/height^2).

~ Solution ~

Step 1: Height^2; 1.9 * 1.9 = 3.46.

Step 2: Weight/height^2; 48/3.46 = 13.9.

Answer: BMI = 13.9.

BMI Example 8

Determine the BMI for a patient who is 1.45 m tall, and has a body mass of 74.5 kg (BMI = mass/height^2).

~ Solution ~

Step 1: The square of the height is 1.45 * 1.45 = 2.1.

Step 2: Mass/height^2; 74.5/2.1 = 35.4.

Answer: BMI = 35.5.

Drug Calculation Workbook

BMI Example 9

Determine the BMI for a 3' 7" tall patient, whose mass is 33.7 kg (BMI = weight/height^2).

~ Solution ~

Step 1: Convert 3 foot to inches; 3 * 12 = 36 inch.

Step 2: Add 7 and 36 = 43 inch.

Step 3: Convert 43 inch to cm; 43 * 2.54 = 109 cm.

Step 4: Convert cm to m; 109/100 = 1.09 m.

Step 5: Square the height; 1.09 * 1.09 = 1.19.

Step 6: Body mass/height^2; 33.7/1.19 = 28.3.

Answer: BMI = 28.3.

BMI Example 10

Determine the BMI for a 68 kg man, with a height of 125 cm (BMI = weight/height^2).

~ Solution ~

Step 1: Convert cm to metres; 125/100 = 1.25.

Step 2: Height^2; 1.25 * 1.25 = 1.5625.

Step 3: Body weight/height^2; 68/1.5625 = 43.5.

Answer: BMI = 43.5.

Body Surface Area

Body Mass Index is not such a good indicator of the dosage requirements for some patients, such as in cardiac and paediatric cases so, instead, the *Body Surface Area* (m^2) is used.

Where a nomogram is unavailable, a calculation must be performed, using one of a variety of methods, with a popular method being the *Mosteller Formula*, where the product of height (cm) and weight (kg) is divided by 3600, and the BSA determined by taking the square root of that calculation.

BSA = Square root of { [height * weight] / 3600 }

Drug Calculation Workbook

Body Surface Area examples

BSA Example 1

Determine the BSA of a patient whose weight is 9.2 kg, and height is 45 cm { sqrt ([height * weight] / 3600) }.

~ Solution ~

Step 1: Multiply weight and height; 45 * 9.2 = 414.

Step 2: Divide 414 by 3,600 = 0.115

Step 3: Take the square root of 0.115 = 0.339.

Answer: BSA = 0.34 m² (square metre).

BSA Example 2

Determine the BSA of a patient whose weight is 99 kg, and height is 1.92 m { sqrt ([height * weight] / 3600) }.

~ Solution ~

Step 1: Convert height to cm; 1.92 * 100 = 192 cm.

Step 2: Weight * height; 99 * 192 = 19,008.

Step 3: 19,008/3,600 = 5.28.

Step 4: Square root of 5.28 = 2.29.

Answer: 2.3 m².

BSA Example 3

Determine the BSA of a patient with a body mass of 54 kg, and a height of 181 cm { sqrt ([height * weight] / 3600) }.

~ Solution ~

Step 1: Weight * height; 54 * 181 = 9,774.

Step 2: Divide 9,774 by 3,600 = 2.715.

Step 3: Take square root of 2.715 = 1.65.

Answer: 1.65 m².

Drug Calculation Workbook

BSA Example 4

Determine the BSA of a patient whose weight is 23 kg, and height of 0.94 m { sqrt ([height * weight] / 3600) }.

~ Solution ~

Step 1: Convert to cm; 0.94 m * 100 = 94 cm.

Step 2: Height * weight; 94 * 23 = 2,162.

Step 3: Divide by 3,600; 2,162/3,600 = 0.6.

Step 4: Square root of 0.6 is 0.77.

Answer: 0.77 m^2.

BSA Example 5

A patient has a BSA of 0.55 m^2, and is prescribed drug A, which is to be administered at a recommended 25 mg per m^2 of BSA, using a stock solution ampoules of 5 mg in 10 ml. What volume of drug A must be administered?

~ Solution ~

Step 1: For a BSA of 1 m², 25 mg will be given.

Step 2: The patient has a BSA of 0.55 m², so should be given 0.55/1 of the supplied 25 mg: 0.55 * 25 = 13.75 mg.

Step 3: Drug A is supplied as 5 mg in 10 ml, therefore, the number of ampoules required is 13.75/5 = 2.75 ampoules.

Step 4: Each ampoule contains 10 ml, which means that 2.75 * 10 = 27.5 ml will be administered.

Answer: 27.5 ml.

BSA Example 6

A patient has a BSA of 0.67 m², and is prescribed drug C, which is to be delivered as 1.2 mg per m² of BSA, using a stock solution of 500 microgram/ml, per ampoule. What volume of drug C must be given to the patient?

~ Solution ~

Step 1: Convert microgram to mg; 500/1,000 = 0.5 mg.

Step 2: If the BSA was 1 m², 1.2 mg drug C would be administered.

Step 3: To deliver 1.2 mg, 1.2/0.5 = 2.4 ampoules of drug C must be used.

Step 4: 2.4 ampoules contains a volume of 2.4 * 1 ml = 2.4 ml.

Step 5: The patient's BSA is only 0.67 m², so only 0.67/1 of the 1 m², dose is required; 0.67 * 2.4 = 1.608 ml.

Answer: 1.6 ml.

BSA Example 7

A patient has a BSA of 0.72 m², and is prescribed drug X, which must be administered as 25 mg/m² of BSA, using a stock solution of 100 mg/10 ml. What mass of drug X must be administered to the patient?

~ Solution ~

The patient's BSA is a 0.72 (72%) fraction of the required 25 mg/m², which is 18 mg.

Answer: 18 mg must be administered.

BSA Example 8

A patient has a BSA of 2.1 m², and is prescribed drug F, which must be delivered as 450 microgram/m², using a stock solution of 2 mg/10 ml. How much drug F, and how many ampoules must be administered to the patient?

~ Solution ~

Step 1: Convert the supplied 2 mg to micrograms; 2 * 1,000 = 2,000 microgram/10 ml.

Step 2: The BSA is 2.1 m², so 2.1 times the supplied 450 microgram = 945 microgram is needed.

Step 3: The number of ampoules needed is 945/2,000 = 0.47.

Step 4: An ampoule contains 10 ml, so 10 * 0.47 = 4.7 ml is the dose.

Answer: 0.47 ampoules, which means 4.7 ml of drug F.

BSA Example 9

A patient has a BSA of 1.8 m², and is prescribed drug B, which must be delivered as 4 mg/m², using supplied 4 mg tablets. How many tablets must the patient take?

~ Solution ~

Step 1: For every square metre of the patient's body surface area, 4 mg (1 tablet) of drug B must be taken by the patient.

Step 2: BSA is 1.8 m², so the dose is 1.8 * 4 = 7.2 mg.

Step 3: To obtain 7.2 mg, tablets required is 7.2/4 = 1.8.

Answer: 1.8 tablets.

BSA Example 10

A patient is prescribed drug Z, at a dose of 5 mg per m^2 BSA. The patient's BSA is 0.8 m^2. Drug Z is supplied in ampoules of 10 mg in 5 ml. What volume of drug Z must be administered?

~ Solution ~

Step 1: The patient needs a 0.8 fraction of the given square metre BSA dose (5 mg/m^2) which is 0.8 * 5 = 4 mg.

Step 2: Drug Z is supplied as 10 mg in 5 ml, so the patient needs four tenths (4/10) of the supply amount; 4/10 * 5 = 2 ml.

Answer: 2 ml.

✦✦✦✦✦✦✦✦✦

Tablet Dosages

The tablet dosage formula is a simple one, it is the prescribed dose divided by the supplied (stock) amount:

> Number of tablets = prescribed dose/supplied dose

Commonly remembered as *what you want / what you have.*

Tablet Dosage Examples

Tablet Example 1

A prescription for 550 mg drug D has been made, and

the available supply is 200 mg tablets. How many tablets should be given?

~ Solution ~

Step 1: Note that he prescribed amount (550) is larger than the supplied amount (200), so the expected answer must be **more** than 1 tablet.

Step 2: Prescribed/supplied is 550/200 = 2.75.

Step 3: The answer meets the expectation that more than 1 tablet is needed, therefore, the numerator/denominator are the correct way around (not inversed).

Answer: **2.75 tablets.**

Tablet Example 2

A patient is to be given 12 g of drug E, supplied in tablets of 30 g each. How many tablets are required?

~ Solution ~

Step 1: The prescribed amount is smaller than the stock amount, so the expected answer will be **less** than 1 tablet.

Step 2: Prescribed/supply is 12/30 = 0.4 (4 tenths).

Step 3: The answer meets the above expectation that the answer is **less** than one tablet, so numerator/denominator are correct.

Answer: 0.4 of a tablet.

Tablet Example 3

A prescription is for 0.45 mg, and the stock supply is 200 microgram. How many tablets are needed?

~ *Solution* ~

Step 1: Convert 0.45 mg to microgram, 0.45 * 1,000 = 450 microgram.

Step 2: 450/200 microgram (prescribed/supply) = 2.25 tablets.

Answer: 2.25 (2 and a quarter) tablets.

Tablet Example 4

A patient requires 4 daily 1.5 microgram doses of drug P, which is supplied in 50 nanogram tablets. What is the total amount of tablets to be taken per day?

~ Solution ~

Step 1: The daily dose is 4 * 1.5 = 6 microgram.

Step 2: In nanograms, 6 * 1,000 = 6,000 nanogram.

Step 3: Prescribed/supply is 6,000/50 nanogram = 120.

Answer: 120 tablets.

Tablet Example 5

To fill a prescription of 1.8 g, using 120 mg tablets, how many tablets will be required?

~ Solution ~

Step 1: Convert the 1.8 g to mg, 1.8 * 1,000 = 1,800 mg.

Step 2: 1,800 takes 1,800/120 = 15 tablets.

Answer: 15 tablets.

Tablet Example 6

A supplied box of drug X contains 40 tablets, providing a total of 9 g. What dose does each tablet hold?

~ Solution ~

Step 1: To make calculation easier, convert the 9 g to mg, 9 * 1,000 = 9,000 mg.

Step 2: The 40 tablets represent a total of 9,000 mg, so each tablets holds 9,000/40 = 225 mg.

Answer: 225 mg per tablet.

Note: If the calculation was made in grams, the answer would be 0.225 g per tablet, which is not as user friendly as using the whole numbers which the milligram calculation does.

Tablet Example 7

From a prescription of 20 mg, the patient has taken 7 tablets with a dose of 800 microgram each. The remaining tablets are 400 microgram each. How many of the remaining tablets should be taken?

~ Solution ~

Step 1: Convert the 20 mg, 20 * 1,000 = 20,000 microgram.

Step 2: Determine how much has already been taken, 7 * 800 = 5,600 microgram.

Step 3: Determine how much remains to be taken, 20,000 − 5,600 = 14,400 microgram.

Step 4: Calculate how many 400 microgram tablets make up 14,400 microgram, 14,400/400 = 36.

Answer: 36 (400 microgram) tablets.

~ Solution ~

Step 1: Convert the 1.8 g to mg, 1.8 * 1,000 = 1,800 mg.

Step 2: 1,800 takes 1,800/120 = 15 tablets.

Answer: 15 tablets.

Tablet Example 6

A supplied box of drug X contains 40 tablets, providing a total of 9 g. What dose does each tablet hold?

~ Solution ~

Step 1: To make calculation easier, convert the 9 g to mg, 9 * 1,000 = 9,000 mg.

Step 2: The 40 tablets represent a total of 9,000 mg, so each tablets holds 9,000/40 = 225 mg.

Answer: 225 mg per tablet.

Note: If the calculation was made in grams, the answer would be 0.225 g per tablet, which is not as user friendly as using the whole numbers which the milligram calculation does.

Tablet Example 7

From a prescription of 20 mg, the patient has taken 7 tablets with a dose of 800 microgram each. The remaining tablets are 400 microgram each. How many of the remaining tablets should be taken?

~ Solution ~

Step 1: Convert the 20 mg, 20 * 1,000 = 20,000 microgram.

Step 2: Determine how much has already been taken, 7 * 800 = 5,600 microgram.

Step 3: Determine how much remains to be taken, 20,000 − 5,600 = 14,400 microgram.

Step 4: Calculate how many 400 microgram tablets make up 14,400 microgram, 14,400/400 = 36.

Answer: 36 (400 microgram) tablets.

Tablet Example 8

The patient has been prescribed 25 tablets of 240 microgram each. What dosage has been prescribed - in mg?

~ *Solution* ~

Step 1: The total dose is 25 * 240 = 6,000 microgram.

Step 2: Convert to mg, 6,000/1,000 = 6 mg.

Answer: 6 mg.

Tablet Example 9

How many 60 mg tablets are needed to make up a prescribed dose of 0.45 g?

~ *Solution* ~

Step 1: Simplify by converting to mg, 0.45 * 1,000 = 450 mg.

Step 2: To reach 450 mg, the tablets required is 450/60

= 7.5.

Answer: 7.5 tablets.

Tablet Example 10

The patient is given 8 tablets of 400 mg each, and a number of tablets of 600 mg each, producing a total of 6 g. How many of the 600 mg tablets has the patient been given?

~ Solution ~

Step 1: The 400 mg tablets total 8 * 400 = 3,200 mg.

Step 2: Convert the total to mg, 6 * 1,000 = 6,000 mg.

Step 3: Determine the amount represented by the 600 mg tablets, 6,000 – 3,200 = 2,800 mg.

Step 4: To make up 2,800 mg, 2,800/600 = 4.67.

Answer: 4.67 (4 and two thirds) 600 mg tablets.

Ampoule Dosages

The above calculation principles, for tablet dosages, can be readily transposed to ampoule (fluid) calculations; where *tablet* becomes *ampoule*, and the terminology of **prescribed dose** and **supply** amount stay the same.

One important issue, which can case confusion, when dealing with liquid solution dosages, is that of the difference between the terms "stock" and "supply", which are often used interchangeably. A drug preparation, which consists of a prescribed amount of a drug or agent, is created from a supplied drug/agent, which is the *supply* amount. The supplied amount, itself, is drawn from stock, which can be described as being a *stock* amount, but these amounts may or may not be the same.

For example, if 20 mg of drug X is to be prepared in an

80 ml saline solution, and drug X is produced, by the pharmaceutical company, as a 100 ml solution containing 50 mg, then the stock, supply, and prescribed values of drug X are:

	Mass	Volume
Stock	50 mg	100 ml
Supply	20 mg	**40 ml**
Prescribed	20 mg	80 ml

Note that the *supply* volume is the volume of the stock solution which contains the prescribed 20 mg, which is a 20/50 = 0.4 fraction of the stock volume, or 0.4 * 100 = **40 ml**. Clearly, stock and supply values can be different.

Drug Calculation Workbook

Ampoule Dosage Examples

Ampoule Example 1

A prescription reads 2.5 million units of drug P, from a supply of ampoules containing 15 million unit/5 ml. What volume should be prepared?

~ *Solution* ~

Step 1: Determine the supply amount per ml, 15 million/5 ml = 3 million/ml.

Step 2: Prescribed/supply is 2.5 million/3 million = 0.83 ml.

Answer: 0.8 ml (rounded).

Ampoule Example 2

The prescription is for 120 mg, from 80 mg/2 ml ampoules. What volume should be drawn up?

~ *Solution* ~

Step 1: Calculate the mass per ml, 80/2 = 40 mg/ml.

Step 2: Prescribed/supply is 120/40 = 3 ml.

Answer: 3 ml.

Ampoule Example 3

A prescription is for 0.6 mg of drug S, from a supply of 50 microgram/ml ampoules, each containing 2 ml. What volume should be drawn up?

~ Solution ~

Step 1: Convert 0.6 mg to 600 microgram.

Step 2: Each ml contains 50 microgram, so prescribed/supply is 600/50 = 12 ml.

Answer: Draw up 12 ml.

Ampoule Example 4

The patient is given 1.2 ml of drug X, from a solution of 1 g in 5 ml. How much drug X has the patient been given?

~ *Solution* ~

Step 1: Convert the supply to mg, 1 g = 1,000 mg.

Step 2: Determine the mass of drug X per ml of solution, 1,000/5 = 200 mg/ml.

Step 2: The 1.2 ml the patient has taken contains the prescribed dose, which is 1.2 * 200 = 240 mg.

Answer: The patient has taken 240 mg.

Ampoule Example 5

The prescription is for 12,000 units, and the supply is 20,000 units in 5 ml. What volume should be drawn up?

~ *Solution* ~

Step 1: Determine the number of units per ml,

20,000/5 = 4,000 units per ml.

Step 2: Calculate prescribed/supply, 12,000/4,000 = 3 ml.

Answer: Draw up 3 ml.

Ampoule Example 6

Drug M is supplied in vials of 0.5 g, and is reconstituted into a solution of 10 ml. If 7 ml is drawn up, how much drug M does that represent?

~ *Solution* ~

Step 1: Convert 0.5 g to mg, 0.5 * 1,000 = 500 mg.

Step 2: Determine the mass of drug M per ml of solution, 500 mg/10 ml = 50 mg/ml.

Step 3: If 7 ml has been drawn up, the mass must be 7 * 50 = 350 mg.

Answer: 350 mg.

Ampoule Example 7

A prescription is for 75 microgram, and the supply is 0.03 mg/ml. What volume should be prepared?

~ Solution ~

Step 1: Convert the supply to the same units as the prescribed amount, 0.03 * 1,000 = 30 microgram/ml.

Step 2: Prescribed/supply is 75/30 = 2.5 ml.

Answer: 2.5 ml.

Ampoule Example 8

A supply of drug T consists of ampoules, each containing 10 mg in 2 ml. A patient needs 0.055 g of drug T. How many ampoules are needed?

~ Solution ~

Step 1: Convert the prescribed amount to common units, 0.055 g * 1,000 = 55 mg.

Step 2: Determine the supply per ml, 10 mg/2 ml = 5 mg/ml.

Step 3: Prescribed/supply is 55 mg/5 mg = 11 ml.

Step 4: Each ampoule contains 2 ml, so 11/2 = 5.5 ampoules.

Answer: 11 ml of drug T, which means 5.5 ampoules.

Ampoule Example 9

A prescription reads 20 mg, from ampoules containing solutions of 75 mg in 5 ml. What volume should be prepared?

~ *Solution* ~

Step 1: Determine the supply amount per ml, 75 mg/5 ml = 15 mg/ml.

Step 2: Prescribed/supply is 20/15 = 1.33 ml.

Answer: 1.3 ml (rounded).

Ampoule Example 10

Drug G is supplied in ampoules of 600 microgram/3 ml. The prescription is for 1.4 mg. How much drug G should be drawn up?

~ Solution ~

Step 1: Convert the prescribed amount to the same units as the supply, 1.4 mg * 1,000 = 1,400 microgram.

Step 3: Determine the supplied amount per ml, 600/3 = 200 microgram/ml.

Step 3: Prescribed/supply is 1,400/200 = 7 ml.

Answer: Draw up 7 ml.

Drip Rates

The set of information needed, to complete a drip rate problem, includes:

- Total volume to infuse
- Giving set drop factor (gtt)
- Drip rate per minute/hour
- Total infusion time, minutes/hours

Drip rate problems might require the answer in terms of volume or drips, either per second, minute, or hour. Consequently, before performing a calculation, the units must be of the same type where, for example, total infusion time must be in minutes, if the drip rate is in minutes.

Drip Rate Examples

Drip Rate Example 1

A patient is prescribed an intravenous infusion, to be given over 3 hours, at a rate of 30 drops per minute, using a giving set with a gtt (drops/ml) of 20. What is the total amount of fluid which will be delivered?

~ *Solution* ~

Step 1: Determine the total drops delivered: 3 (hr) * 60 (min) * 30 (drops) = 5,400 drops.

Step 2: Divide total drops by drops/ml to find the volume delivered: 5,400/20 = 270 ml.

Answer: 270 ml.

Drip Rate Example 2

The iv (intravenous) prescription for a crystalloid, using a giving set with a gtt of 15, states that 25 drops/min should be administered, for a total of 2.5 hours. What is the total amount of fluid which will be delivered?

~ Solution ~

Step 1: Determine the total drops delivered: 2.5 (hr) * 60 (min) * 25 (drops) = 3,750 drops.

Step 2: Divide total drops by drip rate to find the volume delivered: 3,750/15 = 250 ml.

Answer: 250 ml.

Drip Rate Example 3

An instruction is for 0.5 litre of fluid to be given, at a drip rate of 45 drops/min, using a giving set with a gtt of 60. How long will it take to infuse all of the 0.5 litre?

~ Solution ~

Step 1: Convert 0.5 L to ml, 0.5 * 1,000 = 500 ml.

Step 2: Calculate the total drops; 500 (ml) * 60 = 30,00 drops.

Step 3: If 45 drops are delivered per minute, 30,000/45 = 667 minutes.

Step 4: Convert to hours; 667/60 = 11 hours, 7 minutes.

Answer: 500 ml will be infused in 11 hours and 7 minutes.

Drip Rate Example 4

A patient is connected to a giving set, having a drip factor (gtt) of 20, attached to a 1 litre bag of fluid. How long will it take to infuse all of the fluid, if the drip rate is set to 50 drops/min?

~ Solution ~

Step 1: Convert litres to millilitres, 1L = 1,000 ml.

Step 2: Calculate total drops; 1,000 (ml) * 20 = 20,000 drops.

Step 3: Determine how many minutes it takes to deliver 20,000 drops; 20,000/50 (drops/min) = 400 minutes.

Step 4: Convert to hours and minutes; 400/60 = 6

hours, 40 minutes.

Answer: 1 litre will be infused in 6 hours and 40 minutes.

Drip Rate Example 5

A patient is to receive 1 litre of fluid X, over 5 hours, using a giving set with a gtt of 15 drops/ml. What rate, in drops per minute, should be set?

~ Solution ~

Step 1: Total drops to deliver is 1,000 * 15 = 15,000.

Step 2: The 15,000 drops must be delivered over 300 minutes (5 hours), ∴ (therefore) 15,000/300 = 50 drops/min.

Answer: 50 drops/minute.

Drip Rate Example 6

A 250 ml bag of fluid is attached to a blood giving set, which has a gtt of 10. The fluid must be delivered over 2 hours. What drip rate, in drops/min, must be set?

~ Solution ~

Step 1: Calculate the total number of drops; 250 (ml) * 10 (gtt) = 2,500 drops.

Step 2: Convert infusion time to minutes; 2 * 60 = 120 min.

Step 3: Determine drops per minute; 2,500 drops/120 min = 20.83 drops. Rounded to 21.

Answer: 21 drops per minute.

Drip Rate Example 7

500 ml of fluid must be delivered, at a rate of 55 drops/min, using a giving set with a gtt of 20. What volume of fluid will be delivered per hour?

~ Solution ~

Step 1: Determine total drops per hour; 55 * 60 = 3,300 drops.

Step 2: Calculate how many ml are in 3,300 drops; 3,300/20 = 165 ml.

Answer: 165 ml/hour.

Drip Rate Example 8

A giving set, with a gtt of 15, is attached to a 1 litre bag of fluid. If the drip rate is set to 90 drops/min, how much fluid will have been delivered in 45 minutes?

~ Solution ~

Step 1: Determine drops given in 45 min; 45 * 90 = 4,050 drops.

Step 2: Calculate how many ml in 4,050 drops; 4,050/15 = 270 ml.

Answer: 270 ml delivered in 45 minutes.

Drug Calculation Workbook

Drip Rate Example 9

A patient needs an infusion, from a 20 gtt giving set. If the drip rate is set to 120 drops/min, how long will it take to infuse 200 ml?

~ *Solution* ~

Step 1: Determine how many drops in 200 ml; 200 ml * 20 (gtt) = 4,000 drops.

Step 2: Using a drip rate of 120 drips per minute, calculate how lots of 120 drips are in 4,000 drips; 4,000/120 = 33.3.

Answer: 33.3 minutes to deliver 200 ml.

Drip Rate Example 10

Using a giving set with gtt of 15, how much fluid is needed if 75 drops/min are to be delivered, over 40 minutes?

~ *Solution* ~

Step 1: Calculate how many drops will be given in 40 minutes; 75 (drip rate) * 40 (minutes) = 3,000 drops.

Step 2: Convert the number of drops given to volume; 3,000/15 = 200 ml.

Answer: 200 ml will be given in 40 minutes.

❖❖❖❖❖❖❖❖❖

Drug Calculation Workbook

Pumped Infusions

In this chapter, the simplest type of pumped infusion problem is described. For examples of more complex type of problem, refer to ***Pass Your Drug Calculation Test*** *(John England, Amazon)*.

Typical parameters for a flow rate per minute calculation:

- ♣ Total volume to infuse.
- ♣ Infusion time (minutes).
- ♣ Infusion rate (ml/minute).

The precise relationship of the above parameters is given by:

> *Volume infused = infusion rate * infusion time*

OR

Infusion rate = volume infused / infusion time.

Pumped Infusion Examples

Infusion Example 1

An infusion pump must be set to deliver a dose of 450 ml of fluid over 5 hours. What rate, per minute, should the pump be set to?

~ Solution ~

Step 1: In 5 hours, 450 ml will be delivered.

Step 2: In 1 hour, 450 (ml) / 5 (hour) = 90 ml will be delivered.

Step 3: In 1 minute, 90 (ml) / 60 (min) = 1.5 ml will be delivered.

Answer: 1.5 ml/min.

Infusion Example 2

A syringe driver must deliver 50 ml of fluid over 2 hours. How many ml/min should the pump be set to?

~ *Solution* ~

Step 1: In 1 hour, half of the 50 ml will be given: 25 ml.

Step 2: In 1 minute, one sixtieth of the 25 ml will be given: 25/60 = 0.42 ml (rounded).

Answer: Set the driver to deliver 0.42 ml/min.

Infusion Example 3

An infusion pump has to deliver 500 ml of fluid over 4 hours. What infusion rate, per minute, should the pump be set to?

~ *Solution* ~

Step 1: In 1 hour, 500/4 = 125 ml will be given.

Step 2: In 1 minute, 125/60 = 2.1 ml (rounded) will be

given.

Answer: Set the rate to 2.1 ml/min.

Infusion Example 4

A pump is configured to administer 1.6 ml/min. How much fluid will be administered in 3 hours?

~ *Solution* ~

Step 1: In 1 hour, 1.6 * 60 = 96 ml will be given.

Step 2: In 3 hours, 3 * 96 = 288 ml will be given.

Answer: 288 ml.

Infusion Example 5

A pump delivers 12 ml in 15 minutes. How much fluid will be administered in 2 hours?

~ *Solution* ~

Step 1: In 1 hour, 4 * 12 = 48 ml will be given.

Step 2: In 2 hours, 2 * 48 = 96 ml will be given.

Answer: 96 ml.

Infusion Example 6

A patient has received 200 ml of a total 500 ml, from a pump which delivers 1.5 ml/min. If the rate is increased to 2.5 ml/min, what is the total infusion time?

~ *Solution* ~

Step 1: Determine how long it took for the first 200 ml to be administered; 200/1.5 = 133.3 minutes.

Step 2: Determine the remaining volume to be given; 500-200 = 300 ml.

Step 3: If 2.5 ml will be given per minute, calculate how many lots of 2.5 ml (and minutes) are in the remaining 300 ml; 300/2.5 = 120 min.

Drug Calculation Workbook

Step 4: Add the two infusion periods, 133.3 + 120 = 253.3 minutes.

Step 5: Convert to hours; 253.3/60 = 4 hours, 13.3 minutes.

Answer: 4 hours and 13.3 minutes.

Infusion Example 7

At 6 am, a pumped infusion of 1.2 L is commenced, at a rate of 4.5 ml/min. At what time will the infusion be finished?

~ Solution ~

Step 1: Convert litres to ml, 1.2 L * 1,000 = 1,200 ml.

Step 2: Determine how long it will take 1,200 ml to infuse; 1,200/4.5 = 267 minutes.

Step 3: Convert to hours; 267/60 = 4 hours, 27 minutes.

Step 4: Add 4 hours and 27 minutes to 6 am; 10:27 am.

Drug Calculation Workbook

Answer: 10:27 am.

Infusion Example 8

A pumped infusion of 500 ml must be given at a rate of 4.4 ml/min. How long will it take to deliver the 500 ml?

~ Solution ~

Step 1: Determine how many lots of 4.4 ml are in 500 ml, to give the infusion time; 500/4.4 = 113 min.

Step 2: Convert to hours; 113/60 = 1 hour, 53 min.

Answer: 1 hour and 53 minutes.

Infusion Example 9

If a pump is set to deliver fluid at a rate of 1.6 ml/min, how much will be administered in two and a half hours?

~ Solution ~

Step 1: Convert 2.5 hours into minutes; 2 * 60 = 120, plus the 30 minutes = 150 minutes.

Step 2: Calculate the volume which will be delivered in 150 minutes; 150 (min) * 1.6 (ml) = 240 ml.

Answer: 240 ml.

Infusion Example 10

One quarter of a 2 L infusion has been delivered in 80 minutes. What rate, per minute, has the pump been set to?

~ *Solution* ~

Step 1: One quarter of 2 L is 500 ml, so the delivery rate is 500 ml/80 min.

Step 2: Determine the one minute rate; 500/80 = 6.25 ml.

Answer: 6.25 ml/minute.

Displacement Volume

Definition

A specific volume of fluid is displaced when an object, or substance, is placed into a particular space.

In pharmacology, displacement volume is that which is occupied by a drug, when reconstituted with a solvent. For example, if drug Q has a displacement volume of 0.1 ml/50 mg, and 250 mg in 10 ml is to be prepared, then only 9.5 ml of solvent must be added, because the remaining 0.5 ml is the volume displaced by the drug.

Displacement Volume Examples

Displacement Example 1

If it takes 9.6 ml to reconstitute 2 mg of powdered agent X, to a solution of 10 ml, what is the displacement volume, per mg, of X?

~ Solution ~

Step 1: Calculate the volume displaced by the 2 mg of agent X; 10 − 9.6 = 0.4 ml.

Step 2: If the displacement volume is 0.4 ml for 2 mg, then, for 1 mg, the volume must be 0.4/2 = 0.2 ml.

Answer: 0.2 ml/mg.

Displacement Example 2

Calculate the volume of solvent required to produce 1 ml of a 4 mg solution of drug A, the displacement of which is 10 microlitre per mg.

~ Solution ~

Step 1: Determine the displacement for 4 mg of drug A; 4 * 10 microlitre = 40 microlitre.

Step 2: If a solution of 1,000 microlitre (1 ml) is required, and 40 microlitre is provided by the 40 microlitre displacement volume of drug A, then 1,000 − 40 = 960 microlitre are needed.

Answer: 960 microlitre of solvent will reconstitute 4 mg of drug A to a solution of 1 ml.

Displacement Example 3

Drug P, which has a displacement volume 7.5 ml/g, is to be prepared as a 10 ml solution of a 50 mg/ml concentration. How much solvent (water) should be used to reconstitute drug P?

~ Solution ~

Step 1: Calculate how much drug P is needed; For a solution containing 50 mg of drug P per ml, 50 * 10 =

500 mg.

Step 2: Determine the volume displaced by 50 mg of drug P; If 1 gram (1,000 mg) displaces 7.5 ml, then 500 mg must displace 500/1,000 of the 7.5 ml, which is 3.75 ml.

Step 3: Resolve the amount of solvent needed; 10 − 3.75 = 6.25 ml of solvent.

Answer: 6.25 ml.

Displacement Example 4

Drug F has a displacement volume of 1 ml per 30 mg. If 100 mg of drug F should be prepared in a 50 ml solution of WFI (Water For Injections), how much WFI should be used to reconstitute the 100 mg of drug F?

~ *Solution* ~

Step 1: Determine what volume 100 mg displaces; If 30 mg drug F displaces 1 ml, then 100 mg must displace 100/30 = 3.33 * 1 = 3.33 ml.

Drug Calculation Workbook

Step 2: Calculate how much solvent (WFI) is necessary to reconstitute drug F to 50 ml; As 100 mg drug F displaces 3.33 ml, then the remaining volume must be made up with 50 – 3.33 = 46.67 ml.

Answer: Reconstitute 100 mg drug P with 46.67 ml WFI.

Displacement Example 5

Calculate the volume of solvent (0.9% saline) required to produce 5 ml of a 20 mg solution of drug E, the displacement of which is 120 microlitre per 5 mg.

~ Solution ~

Step 1: If 5 mg of drug E produces a displacement of 120 microlitre, then 20 mg must produce 4 (20/5) * 120 = 480 microlitre.

Step 2: Convert the displacement volume to ml; 480/1,000 = 0.48 ml.

Step 3: Determine the volume of solvent to reconstitute

20 mg to a 5 ml solution; 5 − 0.48 = 4.52 ml.

Answer: 4.52 ml of solvent will reconstitute 20 mg of drug E to a 5 ml solution.

Displacement Example 6

Drug M, which has a displacement volume 0.54 ml/g, is to be prepared as a 10 ml solution of a 50 mg/ml concentration. How much solvent should be used to reconstitute drug M?

~ Solution ~

Step 1: To prepare 10 ml of drug M, 50 * 10 = 500 mg will be reconstituted.

Step 2: The displacement volume of drug M is 0.54 ml per g, so, for 500 mg, the displacement will be half (0.5 g/1 g) of the given value of 0.54 ml, which is 0.27 ml.

Step 3: To reconstitute 500 mg of drug M, 10 − 0.27 = 9.73 ml of solvent will be required.

Answer: 9.73 ml.

Displacement Example 7

Drug T has a displacement volume of 450 microlitre per 20 mg. If 50 mg of drug T, in a 20 ml solution, should be prepared, how much WFI (solvent) should be used to reconstitute the 50 mg of drug T?

~ Solution ~

Step 1: If 20 mg has a displacement volume of 450 microlitre, then 50 mg will have 50/20 * 450 = 1,125 microlitre.

Step 2: Convert to ml; 1,125 microlitre / 1,000 = 1.125 ml.

Step 3: As 50 mg drug T produces a displacement volume of 1.125 ml, then the remaining volume will be produced by 20 − 1.125 = 18.875 ml WFI − round up to 18.9 ml.

Answer: Reconstitute 50 mg drug T with 18.9 ml WFI.

Displacement Example 8

50 mg of drug G must be reconstituted into a 10 ml solution. If drug G has a displacement volume of 0.02 ml/mg, how much solvent is needed to produce the required 10 ml solution?

~ Solution ~

Step 1: The total displacement volume, for the prescribed 50 mg of drug G, will be 50 * 0.02 = 1 ml.

Step 2: The remaining volume, for the 10 ml solution, will be formed by the 10 − 1 = 9 ml of solvent.

Answer: 9 ml of solvent is required.

Displacement Example 9

A 100 ml preparation of 5 mg Drug V is prescribed, and the solution is produced with 98 ml of solvent. What is the displacement volume of drug V, per mg?

~ Solution ~

Step 1: Calculate the displacement volume of 5 mg of drug V; The 5 mg has produced 100 − 98 = 2 ml of displacement volume.

Step 2: To determine the displacement volume per mg, divide 2 ml by 5 = 0.4 ml.

Answer: **Drug V displacement volume is 0.4 ml/mg.**

Displacement Example 10

Drug B has a displacement volume of 0.15 ml per 25 mg. 60 mg of drug B, in a 50 ml solution, should be prepared with normal saline (solvent), how much saline should be used to reconstitute the 60 mg of drug B?

~ *Solution* ~

Step 1: Calculate the displacement volume of 60 mg of drug B; 60/25 * 0.15 = 0.36 ml.

Step 2: Determine how much solvent is needed to produce the required 50 ml; 50 − 0.36 = 49.64 ml.

Answer: 49.64 ml.

W/V Drug Concentration

Definition

In pharmacology, concentration describes the ratio of the amount of a drug (solute) to the solution, or excipient, in which it is contained. The most commonly used type of concentration ratio is "mass to volume", which is most often referred to as "weight to volume", and abbreviated to "w/v".

In *Pass Your Drug Calculation Test* (John England, Amazon Publishing), the given advice for calculating w/v problems is based on using a known reference value, and recommends using the 1% w/v concentration (10 mg/ml) of Lidocaine, from which other concentrations may be derived. That advice is continued here.

Terminology

When describing w/v concentrations, using percentages is synonymous with terms in the style of "X in Y". For example, a w/v concentration of 10 mg/ml w/v can be described as **1%** and **1 in 100** solutions.

Weight/Volume Examples

Weight/Volume Example 1

Convert a 3 mg/ml solution to a w/v (weight/volume) concentration.

~ *Solution* ~

Step 1: Using the 1% Lidocaine reference value, where a 1% w/v concentration means 10 mg/ml, the 3 mg/ml concentration represents a 3/10 fraction of the Lidocaine concentration.

Step 1: 3/10 of 1% (Lidocaine w/v) means 0.3%, which is the same as 3 in 1,000.

Answer: 0.3% w/v, or 3 in 1,000.

Weight/Volume Example 2

Drug R is supplied as a solution of 7.5 mg in 20 ml of solvent. What is the w/v concentration?

~ Solution ~

Step 1: If the 7.5 mg was in a 1 ml solution, then it would be 7.5/10 of the 1% Lidocaine reference value, which is 0.75%.

Step 2: Because the given 7.5 mg is in a more diluted solution (20 ml) than the Lidocaine reference volume (1 ml), then the w/v concentration must be 0.75/20 = 0.0375%

Answer: 7.5 mg in 20 ml is a 0.0375% w/v concentration.

Drug Calculation Workbook

Weight/Volume Example 3

What is the w/v concentration of 0.025 g in 5 ml of solution?

~ Solution ~

Step 1: Convert the gram value to milligram; 0.025 * 1,000 = 25 mg.

Step 2: Reduce the concentration value from 5 ml to 1 ml; 25/5 = 5 mg/ml.

Step 3: Compare 5 mg/ml with the 1% Lidocaine reference of 10 mg/ml; 5/10 = 0.5%.

Answer: 25 mg (0.025 g) in 5 ml is 0.5% w/v.

Weight/Volume Example 4

What is the w/v concentration of 80 g in 1 litre of solution?

~ Solution ~

Step 1: Reduce the units from g/L to mg/ml by dividing throughout by 1,000; w/v is 80 mg per ml.

Step 2: Compare the 80 mg/ml concentration with Lidocaine 1% (10 mg); 80/10 of 1% = 8%.

Answer: 80 mg/ml (80 g/litre) is a 8% w/v concentration.

Weight/Volume Example 5

Which is the larger w/v concentration, 25,000 microgram in 5 ml, or 20 mg in 2 ml?

~ *Solution* ~

Step 1: Convert 25,000 microgram to mg; 25,000/1,000 = 25 mg.

Step 2: Determine the concentration of 25 mg/5 ml by converting to a 1 ml value; 25/5 = 5 mg/ml (0.5% w/v).

Step 3: Convert the 20 mg in 2 ml solution to a 1 ml value; 20/2 = 10 mg/ml (1% w/v).

Answer: 20 mg in 2 ml is the larger of the two

Drug Calculation Workbook

concentrations; 1% as opposed to 0.5%.

Weight/Volume Example 6

How many grams of drug X are in 50 ml of a 2.5% solution of drug X?

~ *Solution* ~

Step 1: Derive the 1 ml amount of drug X; compared with 1% Lidocaine, 2.5% is 2.5/1 * 10 = 25 mg/ml.

Step 2: Determine the mass of drug X contained in 50 ml; 50 * 25 = 1,250 mg, or 1.25 g.

Answer: 1.25 g.

Weight/Volume Example 7

Calculate the w/v concentration of 5 g of solute in a 250 ml solution, using normal saline as the solvent.

~ Solution ~

Step 1: Derive the 1 ml concentration; divide 5 g by 250 but, to make calculation easier, firstly convert 5 g to milligrams = 5,000 mg. 5,000 / 250 = 20 mg per ml.

Step 2: Compare 20 mg/ml with Lidocaine 1%, which is 10 mg/ml, or half the concentration of 20 mg/ml.

Step 3: As 20 mg/ml is double the concentration of 1% Lidocaine, then it must be double Lidocaine's 1% value, which is resolves to 2%.

Answer: 5 g in 250 ml is a 2% w/v concentration.

Weight/Volume Example 8

How many mg of solute are contained in 100 ml of a 2.5% w/v solution?

~ Solution ~

Step 1: If 1% Lidocaine is 10 mg/ml, then a 2.5% solution must be 2.5 * 10 = 25 mg/ml.

Step 2: 100 ml of 25 mg/ml is 100 * 25 = 2,500 mg, or

2.5 g.

Answer: 2.5 g of solute.

Weight/Volume Example 9

How much solvent is needed if 60 mg (solute) of a 0.5% w/v solution is to be produced?

~ Solution ~

Step 1: 0.5% is half of the concentration of the 1% Lidocaine reference value, that is, half of 10 mg/ml, or 5 mg/ml.

Step 2: To produce 60 mg, 60/5 = 12 ml is needed.

Answer: 12 ml of 0.5% produces 60 mg solute.

Weight/Volume Example 10

How much of drug X is required if 50 ml of a 1.5%

solution is to be prepared?

~ Solution ~

Step 1: A 1.5% w/v solution contains 1.5 times the amount of solute contained in the 1% Lidocaine reference value, which means 1.5 * 10 = 15 mg/ml.

Step 2: 50 ml of the solution will contain 50 * 15 = 750 mg, or 0.75 g of drug X.

Answer: 750 mg of drug X.

Dilutions

Definition

Supplied drugs are not always constituted in a concentration which is appropriate for a patient, so may have to be diluted to a "weaker" solution. This issue can be likened to diluting a "strong" cup of coffee by adding more water (diluent) – the principles are the same.

Note: The issue of displacement volume is ignored, in the following calculations, for reasons of brevity.

Dilution Examples

Dilution Example 1

Drug B is supplied as 1 ml of a 4% w/v concentration, and must be diluted to 5 mg/ml. How should the final solution be composed?

~ Solution ~

Step 1: Note that our chosen reference value of 1% Lidocaine has a concentration of 10 mg/ml.

Step 2: The supplied solution of drug B is 4%, which is 4 times the w/v concentration of the 1% reference value and, therefore, has 4 times the mass of solute in the same volume, i.e., 4 * 10 mg = 40 mg in 1 ml.

Step 3: The task is to dilute the 40 mg/ml to 5 mg/ml, which is $1/8^{th}$ the concentration.

Step 4: Make up the supplied 40 mg to an 8 ml solution, by adding 7 ml of solvent, giving 40 mg in 8 ml, or 5 mg/ml.

Answer: Add 7 ml solvent to the 1 ml of drug B.

Dilution Example 2

A 10 ml drug C solution, with a 2% w/v concentration, must be used to create 5 ml of a 8 mg/ml solution. Calculate how to produce the prescribed solution.

~ Solution ~

Step 1: Note that 2% is double the concentration of the reference value of 1% Lidocaine, which means drug C is 2 * 10 = 20 mg/ml, giving a total supply of 10 ml * 20 mg = 200 mg.

Step 2: The prescribed 5 ml solution of 8 mg/ml means 5 * 8 = 40 mg of drug C.

Step 3: To extract 40 mg of drug C, from the supplied 200 mg, draw up 40/200 = 1/5 of the supplied 10 ml, which is 2 ml.

Step 4: The remaining volume is made from 5 − 2 = 3 ml of solvent.

Answer: Draw up 2 ml of drug C, and add 3 ml solvent.

Dilution Example 3

A patient requires a 10 ml dose of a 40 mg/ml concentration of drug K, but the only available concentration is 20%, supplied in 5 ml ampoules. How can the prescribed solution be created?

~ Solution ~

Step 1: The patient needs 10 * 40 = 400 mg of drug K, in a 10 ml solution.

Step 2: A 20% w/v concentration means 20 * 10 mg/ml (1% Lidocaine), which is 200 mg/ml.

Step 3: To meet the requirement of 400 mg, 400/200 = 2 ml of the supplied 20% solution are needed.

Step 4: If 2 ml of 20% drug K is drawn up, then another 8 ml of diluent, such as normal saline, must be added, giving a total of 400 mg drug K, in a 10 ml solution, or 40 mg/ml.

Answer: Add 8 ml normal saline to 2 ml of the supplied 20% concentration of drug K.

Dilution Example 4

A 1 ml ampoule of 30 mg/ml drug E must be diluted to a 3 ml solution of a 6 mg/ml concentration. How can this be achieved?

~ Solution ~

Step 1: The target dosage is 3 * 6 = 18 mg of drug E.

Step 2: To extract 18 mg from 1 ml of 30 mg, 18/30 = 0.6 of the supplied 1 ml is needed.

Step 3: Draw up 0.6 ml of the 30 mg/ml ampoule, to produce the required 18 mg of drug E.

Step 4: To make up the remaining volume, add 3 − 0.6 = 2.4 ml of diluent.

Answer: **Draw up 0.6 ml of the supplied ampoule, and add 2.4 ml of, e.g., normal saline.**

Drug Calculation Workbook

Dilution Example 5

Drug M ampoules contain 10 mg in 1 ml of solution. A dilution of drug M is prescribed, with the instruction that 20 ml of a 1 in 2,000 solution is needed. How should this be prepared?

~ Solution ~

Step 1: Determine what 1 in 2,000 means; If 1% Lidocaine, which is 1 in 100, means 10 mg/ml, then 1 in 1,000 must be one tenth the concentration of 10 mg/ml, which is 1 mg/ml.

Step 2: 1 in 2,000 is half the concentration of 1 in 1,000, which is 1 mg/ml, so 1 in 2,000 w/v of must be 0.5 mg/ml.

Step 3: As 20 ml of 0.5 mg/ml are needed, then 20 * 0.5 = 10 mg must be drawn up.

Step 4: Drug M is supplied as 10 mg/ml, which matches the required 10 mg dose, so draw up the 1 ml ampoule of drug M. To make up the required 20 ml, add 19 ml of diluent.

Answer: Draw up all of the 1 ml ampoule of drug

M, and add 19 ml of normal saline (diluent).

Dilution Example 6

A 50 mg dose of drug S must be prepared as a 100 ml solution. How can this be achieved, if 1 ml of 10 mg/ml ampoules of drug S are to be used?

~ Solution ~

Step 1: If 50 mg are needed, 50/10 = 5 of the supplied 1 ml ampoules must be used.

Step 2: To produce the prescribed 100 ml of solution, 100 − 5 = 95 ml of diluent are necessary.

Answer: Draw up 5 of the supplied ampoules, and add 95 ml of normal saline.

Dilution Example 7

Using a supplied 2 ml ampoule, containing 100 microgram of drug F, prepare a solution of 25 microgram drug F in a 5 ml dilution.

~ Solution ~

Step 1: 100 microgram in 2 ml means 50 microgram/ml.

Step 2: The target 25 microgram is 25/50 = 0.5 of the supplied 50 microgram/ml, so 0.5 ml (from the supplied 2 ml ampoule) is needed.

Step 3: Draw up 0.5 ml from the ampoule, and make up the remaining 4.5 ml with normal saline.

Answer: Draw up 0.5 ml of drug F, then add 4.5 ml saline.

Dilution Example 8

A 10 ml solution of a 1 in 10,000 w/v concentration of

drug A is required, but the only available concentration is 0.1%. How should the 10 ml be prepared?

~ *Solution* ~

Step 1: Derive the 1 in 1,000 w/v concentration from the 1% Lidocaine reference; 1%, or 1 in 100, is ten times the concentration of 1 in 1,000, so 1 in 1,000 must be 1/10 of 10 mg/ml, that is, 1 mg/ml.

Step 2: Determine how the supplied 0.1% (1 mg/ml) concentration compares with the required 1 in 10,000 concentration; Obviously, 1 in 10,000 is one tenth the concentration of the supplied 1 in 1,000 concentration, which means one tenth of 1 mg/ml, or 0.1 mg/ml.

Step 3: The re-worded task now is to produce 10 ml of a 0.1 mg/ml (1 in 10,000) concentration, using a 1 mg/ml (1 in 1,000) concentration.

Step 4: 10 ml of 0.1 mg/ml gives 10 * 0.1 = 1 mg in 1 ml.

Step 5: 1 ml of the supplied 0.1% (1 in 1,000) contains 1 mg of drug A, which is the exact mass required. To make the solution up to 10 ml, add 9 ml of solvent to the above 1 ml of 0.1% supply.

Answer: Draw up 1 ml of the 0.1% supply of drug A, and add 9 ml of diluent.

Dilution Example 9

What concentration is formed by adding 2 ml of a 1% w/v concentration of agent X, with 3 ml of a 2% w/v concentration of agent X?

~ *Solution* ~

Step 1: The 1% supply matches the 1% Lidocaine reference value, which is 10 mg/ml.

Step 2: The mass of agent X, contained in 2 ml of the 1% concentration, is 2 * 10 = 20 mg.

Step 3: The 2% supply contains twice the mass, per ml, of 1% Lidocaine, i.e., 2 * 10 mg = 20 mg/ml.

Step 4: The mass of 2% agent X, contained in 3 ml, is 3 * 20 = 60 mg.

Step 5: Add the masses of the 1% and 2% solutions; 20

\+ 60 = 80 mg.

Step 6: Resolve the concentration, per ml; 80 mg in 5 ml of solution means 80/5 = 16 mg/ml.

Answer: The concentration formed is 16 mg/ml.

Dilution Example 10

Create a 20 mg in 5 ml w/v concentration of drug S, using a 2% w/v supply of drug S.

~ Solution ~

Step 1: 20 mg in 5 ml means 20/5 = 4 mg/ml.

Step 2: The 2% supply means 2 times the 1% reference value (Lidocaine), or 2 * 10 = 20 mg/ml.

Step 3: 20 mg/ml is 20/4 = 5 times the concentration of 4 mg/ml. To make the 4 mg/ml concentration, therefore, dilute the 2% supply to a solution which contains 5 times the carrier liquid (diluent).

Step 4: Add 4 ml to 1 ml of the 2% (20 mg/ml) supply

to create a 20 mg in 5 ml solution, as prescribed.

Answer: Add 4 ml of diluent to 1 ml of the 2% supply, to produce a solution of *20 mg in 5 ml.*

Drug Calculation Workbook

Test One

Question 1

Convert 0.0015 g to micrograms.

~ Solution ~

A gram is one million times the value of a microgram, so, multiplying 0.0015 by a million gives 1,500 microgram.

Answer: 1,500 microgram.

Question 2

How many milligrams are there in 0.075 gram?

~ Solution ~

One thousand milligrams comprise one gram, so multiplying 0.075 g by a thousand gives:

Answer: 75 mg.

Question 3

Calculate the Body Mass Index for a patient whose weight is 122 kg, and height is 5 feet 11 inches.

~ Solution ~

Step 1: Write down the formula for BMI: weight / height^2, using kg/m2.

Step 2: Convert 5 feet 11 to inches: (5 * 12) + 11 = 71 inches.

Step 3: Convert 71 inch to cm. 71 * 2.5 = 177.5 cm.

Drug Calculation Workbook

Step 4: Convert 177.5 cm to metres: 177.5/100 = 1.775 m.

Step 5: Square the height; 1.775 * 1.775 = 3.15 m^2.

Step 6: Use the BMI formula: 122/3.15 = 38.73.

Answer: BMI is 38.73.

Question 4

What is the Body Surface Area of a 66 cm child who weighs 30 kg?

~ Solution ~

Step 1: Recall the BSA formula: Square root of { [body weight * height] / 3600}, where weight is in kg, and height is in cm.

Step 2: Weight * height = 30 * 66 cm = 1,980.

Step 3: 1,980/3,600 = 0.55.

Step 4: Square root of 0.55 = 0.74.

Answer: BSA = 0.74 m^2.

Question 5

If a patient is prescribed 1.4 g of drug P, which is supplied in 120 mg tablets, how many tablets are required?

~ Solution ~

Step 1: Convert to a common unit: 1.4 g is 1,400 mg.

Step 2: (Prescribed) 1,400 mg is greater than 120 mg; so the expected answer is more than 1 tablet.

Step 3: Translate the prescribed/supply formula into 1,400/120 mg = 11.67, which meets the expectation that more than 1 tablet is required.

Answer: 11⅔ tablets.

Drug Calculation Workbook

Question 6

A prescription of 900 mg is made for drug A, which is supplied in tablet form, containing 250 mg. How many tablets are needed?

~ *Solution* ~

Step 1: Prescribed (900 mg) is greater than the supplied 250 mg), so the expected answer is more than 1 tablet.

Step 2: Prescribed/supply is 900/250 = 3.6.

Answer: 3.6 tablets.

Question 7

A preparation of drug Q, at 150 microgram per square metre of body area, is required for a patient who weighs 18 kg, and is 60 cm tall. Drug Q is supplied in ampoules with concentration of 50 microgram/ml. How much drug X should be drawn up?

~ Solution ~

Step 1: Declare the BSA formula: Square root of { [body weight * height] / 3600}.

Step 2: Weight * height = 18 * 60 = 1,080.

Step 3: 1,080/3,600 = 0.3.

Step 4: BSA is the square root of 0.3 = 0.55 m².

Step 5: Dose is 0.55 * 150 microgram = 82 microgram. (Note, 82 microgram is greater than the ampoule amount, so more than one ampoule is required.)

Step 6: Ampoules needed: 82/50 = 1.64 (rounded).

Step 7: Volume is 1.64 * 1 ml = 1.64 ml.

Answer: 1.64 ml.

Question 8

A patient, who weighs 74 kg, is prescribed drug Z, 60 microgram/kg/3 times a day, which is supplied in ampoules of 20 mg/5 ml. What total daily volume of drug Z is required?

~ Solution ~

Step 1: A single dose is 74 * 60 = 4,440 microgram = 4.44 mg.

Step 2: The daily dose is 4.44 * 3 = 13.3 mg.

Step 3: Prescribed (13.3 mg) is less than the supply (20 mg), so the expected answer is less than 1 ampoule.

Step 4: Ampoules required: 13.3/20 = 0.67.

Step 5: Each supplied ampoule contains 5 ml, so the volume needed is 0.67 * 5 = 3.3 ml.

Answer: 3.3 ml.

Question 9

How many drops/min are administered, via a giving set having a gtt of 10, if 1.5 L is infused over 3 hours?

~ Solution ~

Step 1: Over 1 hour, 1.5/3 = 0.5 L (500 ml) is given.

Step 2: Drops per hour is 500 * 10 = 5,000 drops.

Step 3: Drops per minute is 5,000/60 = 83⅓.

Answer: 83⅓ drops per minute.

Question 10

If 3 L of fluid is to be administered, via a 15 gtt giving set, what drip rate should be set for a 3 hour infusion.

~ Solution ~

Step 1: In 1 hour 3,000 ml/6 = 500 ml is delivered.

Step 2: In 1 minute, 500/60 = 8.3 ml will be delivered.

Step 3: The number of drips/min is 8.3 * 15 = 125.

Answer: 125 drops per minute.

◊ ◊ ◊ ◊ ◊ ◊ ◊ ◊ ◊

Drug Calculation Workbook

Test two – with answers

The following questions are immediately followed by worked solutions. To complete the test with questions only, skip this section and go to the following *questions only* section.

Question 1

What is the total volume of:

0.48 litre + 7,200 microlitre + 50 millilitre

~ *Solution* ~

Step 1: Convert to a common unit type; 0.48 L is 480 ml,

Drug Calculation Workbook

7,200 microlitre is 7.2 ml.

Step 2: Adding 480 ml, 7.2 ml, 50 ml = 537.2 ml.

Answer: 537.2 ml.

Question 2

Calculate the BMI for a 82 kg patient, whose height is 176 cm.

~ Solution ~

Step 1: Write down the formula for BMI: *Weight/height²*.

Step 2: Convert the height to metres; 176 m / 100 = 1.76 m.

Step 3: Square the height; 1.76 * 1.76 = 3.1 (rounded).

Step 4: 82/3.1 = 26.45/

Answer: BMI is 26.45.

Question 3

A patient needs 2 mg of drug X, per square metre of body surface area. The patient has a weight of 18.8 kg, and height is 72 cm. How much drug X is required?

~ *Solution* ~

Step 1: State the BSA formula; sqrt ([height * weight] / 3600).

Step 2: Multiply weight and height; 72 * 18.8 = 1,354.

Step 3: Divide 1,354 by 3,600 = 0.376.

Step 4: Take the square root of 0.376 = 0.613 m².

Step 5: For 2 mg/m², 2 * 0.613 = 1.23 mg.

Answer: Drug X required is 1.23 mg.

Question 4

A patient is prescribed 480 mg of drug G, which is supplied in ampoules of 50 mg/20 ml. How many drug G ampoules are required, and how much (ml) should be drawn up?

~ Solution ~

Step 1: Determine drug G mass per ml; 50/20 = 2.5 mg/ml.

Step 2: Calculate how much volume will deliver 480 mg; 480/2.5 = 192 ml.

Step 3: How many ampoules is represented by 192 ml? 192/20 = 9.6 ampoules.

Answer: 9.6 ampoules, delivering 192 ml are required.

Question 5

A prescription is for 1,800 microgram drug N, and the available supply is 0.2 mg tablets. How many tablets are needed?

~ Solution ~

Step 1: Convert to a common unit; 0.2 mg * 1,000 = 200 microgram.

Step 2: *Prescribed* divided by *supply* is 1,800/200 = 9 tablets.

Answer: 9 tablets.

Question 6

An intravenous infusion instruction is for 500 ml to be delivered over 90 minutes, using a giving set with a gtt of 20. How many drops per minute should be set?

~ *Solution* ~

Step 1: Determine the total number of drops in 500 ml; 20 * 500 = 10,000 drops.

Step 2: Determine the drops to deliver in 1 minute; 10,000/90 = 111 drops.

Answer: 111 drops/minute.

Question 7

Drug T has a reconstituted displacement volume of 400 microlitre/mg. If 2 mg of drug T is required, in a 4 ml solution, how much solvent is needed?

~ Solution ~

Step 1: Convert 400 microlitre to ml; 400/1,000 = 0.4 ml.

Step 2: As each of the required 2 mg of drug T displaces 0.4 ml, then 2 mg produces a 0.8 ml displacement.

Step 3: Required solution volume is 4 ml, and 0.8 ml of that is the displacement of drug T, therefore 4 − 0.8 = 3.2 ml solvent is needed.

Answer: 3.2 ml solvent.

Question 8

A 10 ml solution of 40 mg/ml of drug B has been prescribed. If the displacement volume of drug B is 3 microlitre/mg, how much solvent is needed?

~ Solution ~

Step 1: mg of drug B needed? 40 * 10 = 400 mg.

Step 2: For each mg of the required 400 mg, a 3 microlitre displacement volume occurs, giving a total displacement of 400 * 3 = 1,200 microlitre.

Step 3: Convert 1,200 microlitre to ml; 1,200/1,000 = 1.2 ml.

Step 4: Of the 10 ml solution, 1.2 ml is the displacement volume, so 10 − 1.2 = 8.8 ml solvent is required.

Answer: 8.8 ml.

Question 9

A 0.5% w/v concentration of drug Z is supplied as a 50 ml solution. How much of drug Z is this?

~ Solution ~

Step 1: Remember the 1% Lidocaine reference value, which is 10 mg/ml.

Step 2: As drug Z is supplied as a 0.5%, w/v, it must be half of the 1% Lidocaine value, which is half of 10 mg/ml, or 5 mg/ml.

Step 3: The are 50 ml of the 5 mg concentration, which means 50 * 5 = 250 mg.

Answer: 250 mg of drug Z.

Question 10

A patient is given 20 ml of a 3% w/v concentration of drug M. How much drug M did the patient receive?

~ *Solution* ~

Step 1: Again, declare the 1% Lidocaine reference value of 10 mg/ml.

Step 2: Drug M has a w/v concentration of 3 * 10 = 30 mg/ml.

Step 3: The patient received 20 ml of the 30 mg/ml solution, which means 20 * 30 = 600 mg.

Answer: The patient received 600 mg of drug M.

◊ ◊ ◊ ◊ ◊ ◊ ◊ ◊ ◊

Drug Calculation Workbook

Test two - questions only

Question 1

What is the total volume of:

0.48 litre + 7,200 microlitre + 50 millilitre

Question 2

Calculate the BMI for a 82 kg patient, whose height is 176 cm.

Question 3

A patient needs 2 mg of drug X, per square metre of body surface area. The patient has a weight of 18.8 kg, and height is 72 cm. How much drug X is required?

Drug Calculation Workbook

Question 4

A patient is prescribed 480 mg of drug G, which is supplied in ampoules of 50 mg/20 ml. How many drug G ampoules are required, and how much (ml) should be drawn up?

Question 5

A prescription is for 1,800 microgram drug N, and the available supply is 0.2 mg tablets. How many tablets are needed?

Question 6

An intravenous infusion instruction is for 500 ml to be delivered over 90 minutes, using a giving set with a gtt of 20. How many drops per minute should be set?

Question 7

Drug T has a reconstituted displacement volume of 400 microlitre/mg. If 2 mg of drug T is required, in a 4 ml solution, how much solvent is needed?

Drug Calculation Workbook

Question 8

A 10 ml solution of 40 mg/ml of drug B has been prescribed. If the displacement volume of drug B is 3 microlitre/mg, how much solvent is needed?

Question 9

A 0.5% w/v concentration of drug Z is supplied as a 50 ml solution. How much of drug Z is this?

Question 10

A patient is given 20 ml of a 3% w/v concentration of drug M. How much drug M did the patient receive?

◊ ◊ ◊ ◊ ◊ ◊ ◊ ◊ ◊

Drug Calculation Workbook

Test Three – with answers

Question 1

The patient has been prescribed 2.5 ml of drug A, from a solution of 0.5 g in 10 ml. How much drug A should the patient receive?

~ Solution ~

Step 1: The prescribed 2.5 ml represents 2.5/10 = 0.25 (a quarter) of the supplied 0.5 g.

Step 2: A quarter of the supplied 0.5 g is 0.125 g.

Answer: 125 mg (0.125 g).

Question 2

Drug B is supplied in 100 mg/5 ml ampoules. A patient, whose weight is 15.5 kg, has been prescribed 4 mg/kg of drug B. How much of drug B should be drawn up?

~ Solution ~

Step 1: Reduce the 100 mg/5 ml to a 1 ml value; 100/5 = 20 mg/ml.

Step 2: The patient needs 4 mg/kg, which is 4 mg * 15.5 = 62 mg.

Step 3: To deliver 62 mg, 62/20 = 3.1 ml are needed.

Answer: 3.1 ml of drug B.

Question 3

Drug C is supplied in 1 ml ampoules of 0.2 mg/ml. The prescribed dose is 20 microgram/kg, and the patient weighs 22 kg. How should drug C be prepared?

~ Solution ~

Step 1: Convert the supply to the same unit as the dose; 0.2 mg * 1,000 = 200 microgram.

Step 2: At a weight of 22 kg, the patient requires 22 * 20 = 440 microgram of drug C.

Step 3: To deliver 440 microgram, 440/200 = 2.2 ml are required.

Answer: 2.2 ml of drug C.

Question 4

How long will it take to deliver an infusion of 250 ml of fluid, using a giving set with a 20 drops/ml drip rate (gtt), and set to 45 drops per minute?

~ Solution ~

Step 1: Calculate the total drops to deliver; 250 * 20 = 5,000 drops.

Step 2: Derive the number of minutes; 5,000/45 = 111 minutes.

Answer: 111 minutes, or 1 hour and 51 minutes.

Question 5

Drug E, with a displacement volume of 240 microlitre/g, must be reconstituted to 12 ml/g. How much solvent is needed if 5 g is prescribed?

~ Solution ~

Step 1: Total displacement volume, for 5 g of drug E, is 5 * 240 = 1,200 microgram, or 1.2 ml.

Step 2: To produce 5 g, 5 * 12 = 60 ml of drug E is required.

Step 3: Solvent needed is 60 − 1.2 = 58.8 ml.

Answer: 58.8 ml of solvent.

Question 6

Drug F has a displacement volume of 16 microlitre per mg. If a solution of 20 mg in 10 ml is prescribed, how much solvent is needed?

~ Solution ~

Step 1: Total displacement, for 20 mg, is 16 * 20 = 320 microlitre.

Step 2: Convert to ml; 320 microlitre divided by 1,000 = 0.32 ml.

Step 3: To fulfil a 10 ml solution, 10 − 0.32 = 9.68 ml of solvent is required.

Answer: 9.7 ml (rounded) of solvent.

Question 7

Convert a 7.5 mg/5 ml solution to a w/v concentration.

~ Solution ~

Step 1: Convert the 5 ml concentration to 1 ml, 7.5/5 =

1.5 mg/ml.

Step 2: Compare 1.5 mg/ml with the 1% Lidocaine reference value of 10 mg/ml; 1.5/10 = 0.15 of 1%, or 0.15%.

Answer: 7.5 mg in 5 ml is 0.15%, w/v.

Question 8

If 20 ml of a 3% solution of drug H is to be prepared, what mass of drug H is required?

~ Solution ~

Step 1: A 3% w/v solution is 3 times the concentration of the 1% Lidocaine reference value, which means 3 times 1% Lidocaine's 10 mg/ml, or 30 mg/ml.

Step 2: As 20 ml of the 3% solution is prescribed, then 20 * 30 = 600 mg is required.

Answer: 600 mg of drug H, in 20 ml.

Question 9

A 2 ml solution of drug K, with a 5% w/v concentration, must be used to dilute the supply to 5 ml dilution of a 5 mg/ml solution. How should the solution be prepared?

~ Solution ~

Step 1: Determine the amount of drug K in 1 ml of the 5% concentration; 5% is 5 times 1% Lidocaine's 10 mg/ml, or 50 mg/ml.

Step 2: 5 ml of 5 mg/ml is required, which means 5 * 5 = 25 mg.

Step 3: 25 mg can be found in 25/50 = 0.5 ml of the supplied 5% concentration.

Step 4: To produce the required 5 ml, add 5 − 0.5 = 4.5 ml of solvent to the 0.5 ml of 5% drug K.

Answer: Add 0.5 ml of 5% drug K to 4.5 ml of solvent.

Question 10

Drug M is supplied as 10 mg in a 1 ml ampoule. Dilute drug M to a w/v concentration of 1 in 2,000.

~ Solution ~

Step 1: The reference concentration of 1% Lidocaine is 10 mg/ml, and can be re-written to "1 in 100".

Step 2: If the dilution was to be 1 in 1,000, then that would be one tenth (100/1,000 = 0.1) the concentration of the above 1% Lidocaine value, which resolves to one tenth of 10 mg/ml, or 1 mg/ml.

Step 3: A 1 in 2,000 solution is half the concentration of 1 in 1,000, so 1 in 2,000 means half of 1 mg/ml, which is 0.5 mg/ml.

Step 4: As the supplied 10 mg/ml of drug M must be diluted to 0.5 mg/ml, then 10/0.5 = 20 ml of solvent is needed.

Step 5: The supplied 10 mg of drug M is in a 1 ml solution, so 20 – 1 = 19 ml solvent is required.

Answer: Add 19 ml solvent to the 1 ml supply.

Drug Calculation Workbook

Test three – questions only

Question 1

The patient has been prescribed 2.5 ml of drug A, from a solution of 0.5 g in 10 ml. How much drug A should the patient receive?

Question 2

Drug B is supplied in 100 mg/5 ml ampoules. A patient, whose weight is 15.5 kg, has been prescribed 4 mg/kg of drug B. How much of drug B should be drawn up?

Question 3

Drug C is supplied in 1 ml ampoules of 0.2 mg/ml. The prescribed dose is 20 microgram/kg, and the patient weighs 22 kg. How should drug C be prepared?

Question 4

How long will it take to deliver an infusion of 250 ml of fluid, using a giving set with a 20 drops/ml drip rate (gtt), and set to 45 drops per minute?

Question 5

Drug E, with a displacement volume of 240 microlitre/g, must be reconstituted to 12 ml/g. How much solvent is needed if 5 g is prescribed?

Question 6

Drug F has a displacement volume of 16 microlitre per mg. If a solution of 20 mg in 10 ml is prescribed, how much solvent is needed?

Question 7

Convert a 7.5 mg/5 ml solution to a w/v concentration.

Question 8

If 20 ml of a 3% solution of drug H is to be prepared,

what mass of drug H is required?

Question 9

A 2 ml solution of drug K, with a 5% w/v concentration, must be used to dilute the supply to 5 ml dilution of a 5 mg/ml solution. How should the solution be prepared?

Question 10

Drug M is supplied as 10 mg in a 1 ml ampoule. Dilute drug M to a w/v concentration of 1 in 2,000.

◊ ◊ ◊ ◊ ◊ ◊ ◊ ◊ ◊

Books by John England

- **Glossary of Anaesthetics**
  http://amzn.eu/g4Ah8AO

- **Q & A: Anaesthetic Principles, Volume 1**
  http://amzn.eu/iIbr8eK

- **Q & A: Basic Life Support**
  http://amzn.eu/acoxDel

- **Perioperative Topics: Test and Learn**
  http://amzn.eu/gMhiDvm

- **Pass Your Drug Calculation Test**
  http://amzn.eu/duk6uT7

- **Basic Drug Calculations**

http://amzn.eu/d0SWtoc

≑ Drug Calculations By Formula
http://amzn.eu/eW9SEg3

≑ Drug Calculation Workbook
http://amzn.eu/d39gtl3

≑ Drug Calculation Examples
http://amzn.eu/6HlGR6Q

≑ Advanced Drug Calculation Workbook
http://amzn.eu/7zDyFQh

≑ Drug Calculation Exercise I
http://amzn.eu/7w117sO

≑ Nurse Q & A: Anatomy and Physiology
http://amzn.eu/f6nRC6G

≑ Q & A: Respiratory System
http://amzn.eu/7RqNNxa

Drug Calculation Workbook

Favourite Quotes

❈ Mathematics is the music of reason. *James Sylvester.*

❈ A farmer counted 197 cows in his field but, when he rounded them up, there were 200 cows. *Anonymous.*

❈ Do not worry about your difficulties in mathematics; I can assure you, mine are greater. *Albert Einstein.*

❈ Without mathematics, there is nothing you can do. Everything around you is mathematics. *Shakuntala Devi.*

❈ In mathematics, you don't understand things. You just get used to them. *Johann von Neumann.*

Printed in Great Britain
by Amazon